OZONE THERAPY
UNABRIDGED

IN LAYMAN'S TERMS
A User's Point of View

BY

ROBERT HATTING

RECENT INFORMATION

The following booklet was written and published in several stages. I'm updating this 10/19 for only one reason: If a reader gleans enough information to further investigate and capture good health again, I've done my job.

I'm a 77-year-old author living in the Philippines writing fiction novels. This is not FICTION! It's the truth as it pertains to my 30-year experience with Ozone Therapy.

Ozone Therapy broke me financially. I lost a ton of money trying to offer my machine and protocols to people in need. It was a lost cause which flushed hundreds of thousands of dollars down the toilet. In addition to the medical and Pharmaceutical industries chastising an threatening me, I had many people cheating me -- a guy traded counterfeit gold coins for a machine, several people just outright took my machines when they had been loaned, and in the Philippines, I actually had two entire systems stolen. One has never been recovered because it's in the hands of terrorists (NPA).

HOWEVER, Healthwise it's been a godsend. It has allowed me to walk again, cured my heart condition without surgery, and cured a debilitating stroke in just a few days. As I mentioned earlier, I'm 77 and have a 34-year-old fiancé. My libido is strong and I'm able to satisfy her needs.

I'm not in the business anymore. I am seeking someone with courage who wants my creations. I'll gift them to the right person.

Original manuscript:

FORWARD

It is very tempting to enlist the aid of some authority figure; a person with many capital letters after his/her name to write this forward. Tempting -- but not in keeping with this manual? Booklet?

Instead I will create a forward by listing my personal uses and observations of people who used this particular therapy and the results they may have received.

MY PERSONAL HISTORY WITH OZONE THERAPY

I took my first Ozone injection from an Ozone Therapy practitioner in Arizona, twenty-four years ago. I had accompanied my riding partner, Rick, to one of his therapy sessions in an attempt to reverse and eliminate his prostate cancer. My friend had been taking these injections for the better part of a month and had experienced excellent results. The ozone generator was a one-of-a-kind custom made in 1957. The unit produced strong and consistent O3.

The practitioner (Doctor Carl) hooked a butterfly needle to a glass syringe and filled the needle and tube with saline solution. He squeezed out some saline to assure there was no ambient air in the needle, disconnected the syringe and capped the tube. He then filled the syringe with OZONE GAS and placed the syringe back on the butterfly needle tube. He inserted the needle into Rick's vein (on the inside of his elbow). He slowly injected the gas into RC's vein. (I was expecting to have to give mouth-to-mouth to my riding partner when I witnessed the gas disappearing into his bloodstream. I wasn't fond of the prospect)

Rick took 75 cc's without batting an eye. This was his twelfth session with Doctor Carl and the dosage was increased each time.

Two days later, I returned with RC and mustered the courage to take 30 cc's — just for grins. (see chapter FOUR for my first major malady)

The injection I received was slightly uncomfortable but not so much that I avoided using this therapy (30 - 60 cc's) to prevent any maladies. A month later the practitioner informed us he no longer had an Ozone generator. The one he had been using was a borrowed unit and the owner needed it returned. By this time Rick had been given a clean bill of health by the medical community — the doctor and the lab. He no longer required extensive treatments, but another patient of the practitioner was mid-way through her cervical cancer treatment.

Rick, Doctor Carl, and I began looking for another Ozone generator. We bought seven different units from various parts of the world over a period of eight months. None of them were satisfactory. The injections and healing capabilities were substandard. RC invested over eight-thousand dollars with a guy who claimed he could build one using the transformer from a neon lighting system. I guess the eight thousand wasn't enough. The clown never produced anything. Meanwhile I was off on one of my adventures to Central America and had the good fortune to run into a former "Share the Wealth" client in the airport in Mexico City. We each had a three-hour layover to catch-up after fifteen years of no contact.

BACKSTORY: At one time Ian and I had worked together to install my performance bonus system (STW)in a company he was running in Seattle. His position as the CEO was specifically orchestrated to 'operate and enhance' the large corporation for its founder who wanted to sell out. The founder and majority stockholder, Peter Brockman, had learned he was suffering from colon cancer. The doctor's prognosis was grim — he had less than a year to live when I arrived on the scene. To shorten the story, I was able to install my system; six months later we had 'dressed up the bride' and I was instrumental in procuring a buyer for the business. Meanwhile, the clock was ticking on Brockman. He left the USA and searched for alternate forms of cancer treatment; first in Mexico and finally Costa Rica. He purchased a nice estate on the coast Costa Rica in Guanacaste province and of course proved everyone wrong by using his genius mind.

Peter had been taking Ozone Therapy from a unlicensed practitioner in Liberia, Costa Rica. The man used a generator that was strong but was still a corona discharge unit. Peter was taking injections every day, so he was experiencing considerable pain because of the unstable effect of straight corona. His genius went to work, and he designed and built the prototype of the machines now being built in Nogales, Mexico — the ones I use. Brockman cured his cancer with the use of his newly designed Ozone Generator. By the time I accidentally ran into Ian at the airport terminal in Mexico City, Brockman had been in business for several years, producing the Ozone generators he credited with saving his life and the lives of countless others. He'd hired Ian to take over the robust business. Ian's mission was to relocate the factory to Mexico; specifically, Nogales on the border with Arizona.

When I asked why the relocation to Nogales from Costa Rica, Ian issued a tirade against the Costa Rican government and their international trade policies.

Not to digress any further, I was able to acquire one of the Brockman designed Ozone Generators. The price back then was $3000.00. It changed my life and actually saved my life years later.

OZONE GENERATORS – an authority?

I am neither an Engineer nor a technician. I'm a user of Ozone Therapy with extensive experience concerning my personal health and those close to me.

Two days ago, a nurse came to my home and with her assistance I was able to inject 55cc of Ozone gas directly into my vein. This is a preventative treatment I take every seven to ten days. I expect to do this treatment for the balance of my life. It's my fountain of youth. At one time (soon after a heart attack) this treatment occurred three times a week and saved my life. Recently a gentleman friend of mine had a stroke and heart attack at the same time. Once he left intensive care and was recovering at home, he began the same treatment. He takes 100 CC's of ozone gas directly into his blood stream --three times a week from an Ozone Generator exactly like the one I own. Nine weeks later, his right-side mobility has returned and his blood pressure has lowered and moderated. The man takes his injections from a machine that provides a smooth painless process. Interestingly, he already had an Ozone generator but when he attempted to take the IV injection, it caused a great deal of pain. WHY? His machine is a weaker model that will only generate O3... never any more molecules. Intermittent O2 molecules are mixed with this weak machine and adds pain to the delivery. In addition, it doesn't provide the healing benefits of concentrated oxygen/ozone. My machine was a major change in his treatment.

These are two examples of many success stories I've either experienced or observed. The treatment is wonderful and very non-invasive. BUT WAIT! --- HOUSTON -- THERE IS A PROBLEM!

Only one company in the world makes this model of Ozone generator – it's located in Nogales, Mexico. The price for each machine is $4,400.00. There is a 2 1/2 year waiting list. 30 months once you pay them a 50% deposit.

The price isn't the major problem; it's the long wait to acquire a machine; the core element in this very effective treatment for a variety of ills. Shoot, I know people who would pay twice the sticker price to get one on a timely basis. *When one is dying of cancer or a heart condition a few thousand dollars doesn't seem like much when you know it will cure you...*

Recently, I was able to purchase some parts from a Brockman designed machine. I sent these parts to my friend in Vancouver, BC. He has a firm that reverse engineers products; specifically, electronics. He then forwards his findings to his staff in Singapore. JJ was about to leave to spend the winter in Asia, so I was fortunate he started the project before left on his journey.

REVERSE ENGINEERING

I received word this morning that JJ, my guy in Vancouver, BC has just arrived at his office in Singapore. His initial findings have encouraged me to take the next step. I forwarded the cash to pay his initial fee for the initial appraisal of the system he is re-engineering.

On our Skype call, JJ related some of his technical findings and discoursed on how he was approaching the replication. I listened politely and nodded or smiled at the pauses I thought were appropriate. The truth of the matter is: I don't care how he achieves the concentrated ozone molecules. I'm only interested in results. If I can inject 50 or 100 cc's of the concentrated ozone gas into my veins without discomfort, he has accomplished his mission.

Assuming we're successful, the next steps are a collaboration between Myself, JJ, and whoever we choose to manufacture the units/parts. Once this phase is accomplished, JJ's role as a consultant is over and I will own a prototype product; the nucleus of a business opportunity. My past experience in business suggests that this opportunity will be as small or as large as I choose it to be. Now it's time to reflect, contemplate, and make a plan.

PERSONAL EXPERIENCES

Between the time we lost our Ozone machine and the one I finally acquired from the Brockman factory in Nogales, Rick and I went through a variety of Ozone generators. Doctor Carl borrowed and bought a few as well. Once the Brockman machine entered our lives, we stopped looking. The factory in Nogales made two models. The strong one for IV injections and a less powerful unit for ozonating water and olive oil. Since RC and I were making fairly good money in other ventures, we co-purchased a strong unit for Doctor Carl. He was elated and so were his patients. Most of the sub-standard units we purchased were used to purify water in the horse troughs. In a couple of tanks, we had to replace them with Brockman's second level unit. The substandard "medical units" couldn't keep down the algae in a horse trough. I finally found a source for the 'horse trough' units — the best ones for the money came from Taiwan. We actually devised a unit to run off a 12-volt motorcycle battery and a small solar panel. Those units serviced several remote water tanks for RC's cattle.

When I was traveling extensively to Costa Rica and Panama. I ran across a fellow who operated a botanical garden. I bought a machine (the $3000 strong one and told him it was $1500. He paid me the $1500 and immediately buggered it up (or his son did) I bought another for a replacement. I took the damaged unit back to the factory and they couldn't issue me any credit because the inside of the tube was contaminated. (I learned later that they had used oxygen from their oxygen/acetylene system — the same regulator and hose) UGGGH!! I returned later with proper tubing, a medical regulator, and a glass syringe. I also brought down a machine for a friend. It was damaged during shipping, so I never collected. That was a very costly trip.

During the time I was traveling around; being a good Samaritan, RC and Doctor Carl were treating people with serious conditions; from Cancer & AIDS on one end of the spectrum to various non-life-threatening maladies including herpes, diabetes, chromes disease, ulcers, and skin cancer on the other. RC applied several treatments on his horses to cure equine maladies; including cancer, fistula withers, hernias, and various stages of lameness. He treated several cows and calves that were suffering from a tick fever found often in arid climes like southern Arizona. He treated them with IV injections, just like he'd received for his prostate cancer.

Rick's cattle herd experienced a higher than usual calf crop by maintaining ozonators in the water troughs. Clean water seemed to enhance the overall health of his cattle. (this condition is still the same. His calf crop is 15% higher than pre-Ozone.)

Book tour, 2006 — THE MIRACLE

For almost 7 months, I was on a book tour with various authors including Michael Blake. Less than a year prior, I couldn't conceive of performing the task required to do all that traveling and activity. I was confined to a roll-around-chair from a serious accident I had had with a horse. I was told by two doctors that I would never walk again. Correct that; two doctors in two different hospitals.

Instead of driving to the store that sold wheelchairs as the last doctor had suggested, RC drove me to see Doctor Carl.

Carl looked at the x-rays, and then at my body which was totally black from my waist to mid thighs — on both sides. Even my penis was totally black. X-rays showed my pelvis was shattered like an egg (13 pieces) and my tail bone was fractured. All my muscles, tendons and ligaments were either torn or highly bruised.

Doctor Carl began IV injections of Ozone. I took a 100-cc injection once a day for seven days. Then I took four injections a week and a few weeks later the therapy was reduced to three times a week. Six weeks later I was walking without crutches and assistance, but I was still taking two injections a week. My walking was not a normal walk for me but more of a forward shuffle in an upright position. Looking back, I should have remained and completed another six weeks of therapy, but I was anxious to return to Central America; specifically, Panama and Costa Rica.

I lived a rather sedentary life while in Costa Rica and Panama. It pained me to walk any distance (it still does) and I gained weight because of minimal exercise. I returned to Arizona and started the book tour six months to the day from my first step without crutches. I wasn't in top shape, but I wasn't an invalid, either. Unfortunately, I didn't continue with the Ozone therapy. I was too busy peddling my novel, PARTNERS; traveling most of the lower forty-eight states. Following the book tour, I picked up my new Brockman Ozone Generator and flew back to Panama. Everything had been moved off the boat and in had been stored. I rented a house, bought some furniture, and began treating a Panamanian lady friend with ozone therapy. She suffered from acute Chromes disease. In six weeks, she was back to eating normal and showed no signs of the disease. That was later confirmed by a blood test and exam at one of the local clinics. My friend went away a happy camper.

Shortly after she was finished with her treatments, I moved to another rental house. During this move, I returned the medical oxygen tank and placed my Ozone Generator in the closet. I didn't use it for 3 years.

OOPS! What's that pain?

Life is full of decisions and consequences. I had a $4,400.00 ozone Generator in the closet, and I wasn't using it. Not even for cleansing my water. I was feeling good right up until I felt this sever pain in my chest. Wow — that was a scrotum squeezer! I knew it was the end for me. I drove myself to the hospital, dicked around with those idiots for the better part of a day only to confirm what I already knew. I was having a heart attack. The details are almost comical — I won't bore you with them. However, their facilities, incompetence, and the expense of a triple bypass operation pushed me in another direction. I had two choices as I saw it: #1 drive to the beach and try to swim to Hawaii. #2 drag out the Ozone generator, order a tank of Oxygen and get with the program. I called Doctor Carl and gave him an overview of my problem. He prescribed my treatment via phone calls. I enlisted the aid of a local doctor to help me by monitoring my condition — keeping the meds prescribed and even making house calls to check my Blood Pressure. I hired a technician to come to my house and administer the ozone gas by inserting the needle into my vein. This happened every day or a week and then we tapered off to three times a week for nine weeks. By the end of the 3rd week, my blood pressure had stabilized, and I was able to cut the prescribed pills in half. Also, at that time I noticed a major change in my libido. More about that later...

By the end of the 4th month, I was only taking one-half of the blood pressure pill a week. By the sixth month I was taking one injection per week and NO MEDICATION! None — nada — zip!

A short return to the past.

A week before my heart attack, I had my eyes examined. I was informed I had a cataract forming on my right eye. I bought some new lenses (with really cheap frames) in order to compensate for this temporary condition. Six years prior I had a similar condition forming on my left eye. Using ozonated water and an eye cup, I was able to reverse the process in several weeks. I was sidetracked with my heart attack and didn't revert back to the eye therapy until three weeks after the cardiovascular therapy began. By the time I was off the meds I was also seeing better. I returned to the eye doctor and shocked her with my announcement. She reexamined, confirmed the cataract was gone, and re-prescribed weaker lenses.

A GOOD FRIEND owns a fishing resort some distance from David. Nine months after my heart attack, I took a lady friend to his resort for Xmas dinner. He was shocked and pleasantly surprised at my success story. He then admitted that he was having some serious prostate problems. In fact, he was wearing a catheter as we spoke. Later I learned he had blood showing in this catheter. He began making the 2 1/2-hour trip to visit me three times a week and was eventually cured of his prostrate condition using IV Ozone injections. He comes to town periodically and usually arranges to have a 55-cc maintenance injection.

During this same time period several people rented my machine to deal with a variety of conditions. Most were successful. A few were not. Most of the failures were one treatment and no follow-up. It was about this time I became worried; "What happens if my machine breaks?" I'd never considered the longevity of the unit until my life and well-being was dependent on the therapy. I made a call to my friend RC in AZ and spoke with him about my concerns. He suggested I relieve my concern by using one of our "Horse Trough" units for ozonating water and olive oil — to save the Brockman designed unit for medical only.

I knew his logic was sound, but I really wanted another machine to back mine up. I ordered the parts for the 'horse-trough', a strong corona discharge unit. Our supplier in Taiwan sold it to me for $265. By the time it arrived in David, Panama, I had almost $400.00 invested in the parts and it still needed assembly. I set about creating my alternate generator by installing it in an old toolbox. I ordered the hose and some fittings from an industrial warehouse in the states and soon the unit was bubbling my water and olive oil.

BACK UP UNIT

My message to Doctor Carl concerning the back-up unit was heard loud and clear but my nagging for a better position on the list went unnoticed because Peter Brockman had died eight years prior at the age of 89 and my old friend Ian had recently retired. The management was in the hands of the Mexican employees — now owners. Brockman and Ian had set it up so the factory workers and managers were the recipients of the business; a Mexican ESOP if you will. I tracked down Ian and finally had a message delivered just before he moved to Europe. He arranged for Doctor Carl to be placed on the list; near the top. I sent money through RC to make my 50% deposit and then waited and waited. Five months. This was two years to the day I had suffered the heart attack.

In the meantime, I was using the horse-trough generator to keep my water supply ozonated and occasionally I would use it to do Ozonated Olive Oil. A user needed OOO to handle a parasite condition. Just a small amount of OOO requires 30 minutes in three increments...minimum. The user complained about the volume and price. I showed them the door!

The day finally arrived that I was the proud owner of another Brockman designed Ozone generator. I paid the balance of my purchase price and RC drove to Nogales from his ranch near Tucson to pick it up. Now I had 2 Brockman's and the Horse machine. A total of almost ten thousand dollars invested in Ozone generators. One of them was sitting in a ranch house in the Arizona desert, so I booked a flight to Tucson. I wanted to hand carry my new unit back to David.

I delayed the trip twice for a variety of reasons and finally had the unit shipped to me. The transportation cost exceeded the cost of my Horse Trough generator.

A VOICE FROM THE PAST;

Having the second machine in my house was a big relief. I was open again to others using my machine. I didn't make any announcements, but several people heard I was renting my machine again and came for some help.

One woman showed up at 5 o'clock one morning with a horrible back-story. I knew her slightly — she was the wife of a Canadian man who fathered her three kids and then left her to fend for herself while he was off in Quebec with his mistress. He returned a year later and wanted to assume his husbandly role. He gave her a dose of herpes as a return gift. She went to the Regional Government Hospital and condition was diagnosed with an exam and blood test. She needed a miracle. She had divorced the Canadian guy but knew she could never marry again in Panama with the STD on her record.

I had her obtain another blood test at an independent lab. Sure, enough it was positive for herpes Simplex 2. She began vaginal insufflations. Twenty -- fifteen-minute treatments plus Ozonated Olive Oil for topical application. At the end of three months she went to another independent lab and tested negative for the STD. I sent her to another private hospital lab for another blood test. She took those two negative blood tests back to the regional officials and claimed they had made a mistake. She was retested again. Three independent tests showed she was negative, so her records were changed.

The peace of mind of having the second machine was exhilarating for several months until it dawned on me as I was packing for my ticketed flight to the US, that having the back-up machine in the same room with my primary machine was foolhardy because if a thief broke into my home while I was away, they would take both units. (*I have had 2 home invasions since moving to Panama — I'm an experienced victim!*)

So, I took one of the units and loaned it to my friend out on the peninsula. He attempted to find a person to administer his injections but to no avail. He brought the unit back and I rented it to a lady in Boquete who was suffering from ovarian cysts. She used it while I was back in the US and solved her problem. The journey to Arizona was quick (10 days) but I was able to accomplish most of my scheduled tasks; including an exam by Doctor Carl.

I was deemed the Poster Boy for Ozone Therapy by doctor Carl. He had my original EKG; the blood test results and of course had monitored me along my road to recovery. His physical exam indicated I still suffered problems in the pelvic and lower back — a condition I knew would not resolve itself in this lifetime. However, my heart attack recovery showed no serious problems. I would always have a limited physical stamina because of my heart damage and my continuing pelvic problems. However, my cardiovascular system was that of a 50 year old triathlon athlete. That accounts for my mental stamina. My day usually starts at 4 am and ends around 9-10 in the evening. I was thrilled to hear that my self-administered technique was successful.

I returned to Panama with the knowledge that my method of medical treatment was sound and not just a fluke.

Panama is the repository for every con artist and charlatan in the world. Many so-called alternative healing practitioners have moved down here and have begun scamming the populace; selling or using ozone generators that produce less than my Horse Trough unit. Other folks set themselves up as experts and have actually given Ozone therapy a bad reputation — absolutely no results for the dollars spent.

I listened to the negative remarks, read the scathing reports on the chat rooms and adjusted my attitude toward the gringo population here in Panama. (most are narcissistic idiots). I found a natural healing clinic in Bella Vista and sold my older Brockman Ozone generator to them with the agreement they would be my back-up. Their primary nurse had studied Ozone Therapy and has come a long way in treating various patients. I instructed her on giving IV injections and she is now offering that as one of her services. She is able to perform at a high level because she uses the best machine ever produced in the world. She has witnessed miraculous-like results from her treatments.

HERE COMES A NEW POSTER BOY!

An acquaintance of mine, called and wanted an ozone injection. He was having trouble sleeping and he lacked energy. He drove the hour and fifteen minute trip to be at my house but the nurse I had scheduled for the injection never showed up — she didn't call, nothing! (typical behavior for Panama). It was a bust and the nurse has never been called back. That following weekend, my friend had a stroke and a heart attack — at the same time. I visited him in Intensive care, his condition was serious. They had to put in a stint and his entire right side suffered from paralysis. He was allowed to return home after spending a week in the intensive care unit but then was re-admitted a few days later. I visited him often and we discussed his future health. He wanted to use the Ozone therapy to remove the blockages so he wouldn't have to have another stint implanted.

This man already owned an ozone machine. He used it mostly for ozonating water. I discovered later he was sold a bill of goods by one of the quack practitioners. More on that later. It had a lot of dials. I asked what they were for... he answered that it was to regulate the oxygen in — and the ozone out.

<u>WHY WOULD ANYONE WANT LESS OZONE FROM AN OZONE GENERATOR?</u> *(MY MACHINE IS SET TO PRODUCE THE STRONGEST OZONE! YOU REGULATE THE FLOW WITH THE REGULATOR ON THE OXYGEN TANK!)*

MY MAN began his IV injections two weeks out of the hospital. Doctor Carl was apprised of his condition and prescribed the treatment. I drove to his home to treat him with my machine and then afterward he drove to mine for a couple of weeks to get his injection. MY MAN ordered several glass syringes and was finally able to take his IV treatment closer to his home — with the back-up machine I sold MY NURSE. She administers the injections three times a week as prescribed by Doctor Carl. I'm pleased to report that MY MAN has recovered his right-side mobility and feeling. (He is out driving his car and sometimes his motorcycle.) He has controlled his blood pressure and reduced his dependency on the pills prescribed by the medicos. MY MAN is a true believer 10/23/19 – *HE JUST TURNED 80).* He understands the difference in Ozone generators. He and MY NURSE are a team of cheerleaders. MY NURSE has become in demand all of a sudden. This is wonderful but also scary... *What happens if her machine breaks — the back-up to mine?* **What if?** The worry warts begin to emerge at a time I cannot afford another machine. Nor is one available. THIRTY-TWO months and $4400.00 is what the Nogales people quoted my friend, RC a couple of weeks ago.

RANCHER RICK TO THE RESCUE

RC sold a rope horse to one of the employees of the Nogales ozone factory; one that lives on the US side of the border.

I got lucky because of this connection.

The roper/employee was able to procure the innards of a Brockman designed Ozone Generator. He sold them to Rick for $2900.00. RC in turn liquidated our rodeo stock fund to reimburse himself and was ready to ship the parts to me here in Panama. My plan was to make a back-up unit and keep it somewhere safe. Then I began to think about the future. I suspected that soon, we would be arriving at the same point as now — dependent on a machine we couldn't acquire for 30+ months. Since both machines were operating without problems, I decided to gamble my new parts.

Many years ago, I had learned that Peter Brockman refused to patent his Ozone invention because of what happened to him with his laser cutter business. (he was knocked off immediately after the patent was filed. He didn't want that to happen to the Ozone generator so instead of the patent, every employee privy to the SECRET had to sign a non-disclosure agreement.)

Like I said — I opted to gamble. I instructed RC to send the parts to a mutual friend in Vancouver BC.

JJ has a very thriving business doing reverse engineering. He is also the owner of a Brockman designed Ozone Generator. (Doctor Carl treated him for Colon cancer 8 years ago.) JJ understands the needs and results as well as anyone. He was pleased to reduce his fee to do his specialized magic. He used the equipment in his Vancouver lab to re-engineer the parts and sent the results to his facility in Shanghai. He was scheduled to spend the winter in Asia like he does every year. He was so confident he could replicate the Brockman design; he left his Nogales Ozone machine with his brother in Vancouver, BC.

JJ and I have been communicating every day concerning his progress. JJ had to fly to Jakarta and told me to look for a letter from his secretary. It arrived a couple of days ago. She informed me of a fed-ex package headed my way. I check the tracking number every day. JJ has assured me he took an injection with reassembled and acquired components and that it was 'equal to -- or better than' the Nogales machine. That is good news. I have ordered a full complement of assembly parts; cords, switches wiring, fittings, norprene and silicone tubing, plus I've designed a special box for the unit to be housed.

Within a couple of weeks, I expect to prove to myself if the new components are comparable to the Nogales units. If they are, it's good news to the world of Ozone therapy. Especially those of us who are dependent on the prime medical generators for our healthy lives.

NOT A MAGIC BULLET

It needs to be noted and understood that Ozone therapy with the Brockman design or my new unit (do I need a name?) is not a magic bullet. One needs the correct application, a careful regimen of a complimentary diet, exercise, and precaution to minimize the causes of the origin of the malady. Given these parameters, adding extra oxygen to your bloodstream will definitely improve whatever condition that is affecting your overall health. The body becomes the director of the healing process. Strange as it may seem, once you add the concentrated oxygen into your bloodstream, you can't will it to go to a particular organ or malady. The body is going to address whatever is the most serious condition that exists. (a condition that you may not know exists)

A gentleman from Boquete heard about my machine and came to me because his PSA score was very high. He was certain he was getting prostate cancer. He was injected for several weeks under the guidance of Doctor Carl. He went and had his PSA tested after 3 weeks. It was higher than before. However, his skin cancer had disappeared. He went to another type of therapy for his prostate. I have no idea if he resolved the prostate problem, but his body used the ozone therapy to cure his skin cancer.

LIBIDO
There is a side-effect to taking IV injections of Ozone gas. The circulatory system returns to its youth and so does a man's libido.

I can't see why this is a negative side effect. Some may consider it bad, but I suspect it will not be the men experiencing this 'fountain of youth' phenomenon. Just speaking for those who have been forthright with me. *This is not just morning wood. This is the libido of our forties!*

Only one of the ladies has spoken on this topic; the woman who had been cured of the herpes. She informed me of a heightened sexual awareness during and after her treatments. She volunteered this information midway through her treatments and again after she received her clean bill of health. I've not asked any of the other female users. It would be bad form.

USE YOUR common sense. Some foods and drink will kill you over time. Everyone knows these truths in a general sense, but one has to have had a major health scare to really pay attention.

Salt & sodium will hurt my system — just like any other poison. Now that my body is a fine-tuned healing machine, it detects the poisons in food and drink. You can't fool it with a label on a box that says zero grams of sodium. My body knows. The food processor lied...not my body. Pay attention to these signs once you begin Ozone therapy. You will soon have a list of liars and forbidden items.

CHAPTER 1a

This addition (addendum)to the booklet you are reading has been compiled over the past two years since the first version was published in December of 2103. I was living in Panama at the time I created my first ozone generator using my new technology to enhance a straight corona discharge and make it a double phase similar to the Brockman generators of Nogales, Mexico.

When I created the crystal modulator in the summer of 2013, I had to cash in my retirement reserves to pay for the engineering and tooling for my invention. I felt very strongly about offering a medical miracle to the masses. Unfortunately, my intentions were soon being questioned and sometimes scorned. My costs for each unit were enormous because of the low volume of component purchases. Everything was custom, and even the simplest parts for assembly could not be found in Panama.

The first unit constructed in my home in David, Panama, was housed in a hardwood box. It was tested several times on myself and then used in an ozone center in Bella Vista, Chiriqui. In search of another material for the housing, I chose aluminum. My first design was heavy and difficult to assemble. The Panamanian aluminum welders couldn't grasp the concept that the case was for a quasi-medical instrument.

The first three units were sold but later the cases were replaced for the Phase two design; a simple rectangular case measuring nine inches tall by nine inches wide by fifteen inches deep._ As the exterior case was being redesigned, so were the inner workings of the unit. To date, there have been four major evolutions to the invention; becoming a double duty ceramic tube powered by a unique and customized power supply. The results are the same; 03,06,09, and sometimes 012.

These redesigns have created a smaller footprint and a more reliable assembly process. I still modify each unit and check each one for quality before they are used or shipped. To lower the cost, I now have my cases made in Taiwan, the innards made in three different countries with the wiring completed in Taiwan, and final assembly done in the Philippines. Since I am now residing in the Philippines, the costs have been lowered substantially.

CHAPTER 2a

BREATHING APPARATUS: For the lack of a more descriptive name, my invention
will be referred to as Breathing Apparatus or
BA.

This is an adjunct to my ozone generator that allows a user to breathe ozone directly from the ozone generator. Let me explain how important this and how this came about.

Years ago, in a telephone conversation with Peter Brockman, the creator of the double stage medical grade ozone machine, he corrected me when, out of ignorance, I referred to the noxious smell of ozone. In a polite, but stern, manner he lectured me on the erroneous conceptions that all the experts seem to parrot about the smell of ozone. Brockman told me that ozone has no smell, color or taste. Ozone (O_3) is concentrated oxygen molecules — how can it have a smell? He further explained that when ozone hits the ambient air it creates many elements, but the predominant toxic form is Nitric Acid (HNO_3). That's what you smell when lightning strikes the atmosphere and creates ozone: the nitric acid created when nitrogen and hydrogen combine with three molecules of oxygen.

So, recalling this conversation in my mind from several decades prior, I decided to find a way to neutralize the nitric acid and still allow the Highgrade ozone become available to breathe. Many, many hours and many failures later, I discovered that certain precious metals combined with other ingredients will indeed allow one to breathe ozone, provided the user's lungs become the pump to pull the gas through the apparatus and not let the concentrated ozone reach the ambient air. It has been used by several hundred clients in ozone centers, plus those in private systems, including myself. I'm able to take my ozone therapy without injections.

Of all the protocols, this BA is perhaps the best ratio of non-invasive to performance I have encountered. I still believe the Direct Injection (DI) is the most positive method for both genders to cure a serious malady like cancer, a heart condition, or a stroke. However, dealing with less life-threatening conditions makes the BA a star of the protocols. No fuss, no pain, and no technician needed. Just hang on the mask and breathe deeply for ten minutes. (The male libido also responds to this protocol)

One of the issues facing anyone who has used a medical grade ozone generator is obtaining oxygen. Most North American and European countries require a prescription from a doctor to acquire a tank of medical oxygen. The BA works perfectly with a mid-grade oxygen concentrator. Dialed back to the lowest settings, most oxygen concentrators generate ninety percent oxygen (90%), which is more than sufficient to operate the BA and do most other protocols. (I still recommend 100% medical oxygen for direct injections.)

A couple of ozone centers now have a small tank of oxygen and a regulator they use for direct injections and an oxygen concentrator they use for all other protocols; water, oils, virginals, and the Breathing Apparatus. It has saved them money and the hassle of dealing with refilling tanks.

I'm proud of my double stage ozone generator that produces 06,09, and sometime 012, but I'm triple proud of my Breathing Apparatus. This invention really changes the complexion of ozone therapy.

CHAPTER 3a

This chapter is primarily a How To: nothing tricky or revolutionary. Just keep in mind that the protocols used on my system will not apply equally to other ozone generators on the market.

WATER — the ozonation of water depends on the size of the   bottle. (ALWAYS USE GLASS OR STAINLESS STEEL — never plastic or aluminum.) I always use one-liter glass bottles and ozonate them for 30 seconds to purify the H_2O. Water for medicinal purposes should be twice that time - one minute per liter. But it should be chilled first to hold its healing qualities. Forty- to fifty degree water will hold the ozone for about six to eight hours if refrigerated. It's still good to drink after that time because it's really purified and may at times hold a bit of healing power, but most of the healing properties will have dissipated after six hours.

OILS - Most oils will hold the ozone healing powers for a week to ten days. Choosing which one is based on preference. I've read that olive oil holds the ozone the longest. You know me - I set out to test what the so-called experts say which proved to be <u>bovine excrement!</u> My testing proved palm oil and coconut oil actually held the healing properties longer than olive oil, especially when refrigerated. Ozonating honey is a bit more complicated, but it works great to give to children who suffer the runny noses and other minor maladies. One has to heat the honey to raise the viscosity before bubbling ozone gas. I've been ozonating all the oils and the honey for five minutes per four ounces. My personal preference for ingestion is coconut oil because the taste is better. Most ladies use the ozonated coconut oil to remove their makeup and have found they are also removing some wrinkles. My friend Linda suggests using ozonated coconut oil mixed with baking soda for a deep cleaner.

BREATHING APPARATUS — No one else has one so don't look for guidance from the Internet or medical experts. Unless some doctor has used the OLD TREE Ozone system — the 06-model ozone generator plus my exclusive breathing apparatus - they are speaking out of their ass! No one knows anything — except those of us who use the system. I have witnessed the results firsthand — especially in the prevention and virility side of this equation. Unless one is suffering a serious malady, ten minutes a day on the breathing apparatus will improve overall health, increase energy levels, and put lead in a guy's pencil. It is the least invasive method to get men to try and use ozone therapy. Ladies have most success with vaginals but also like the breathing apparatus because it enhances their normal routines.

DIRECT INJECTION — Absolutely the fastest protocol to cure a malady or prevent medical problems such as: Cancer, Heart Conditions, Strokes, STD's (including AIDS & HIV) Diabetes, Erectile Dysfunction, Multiple Sclerosis, Hepatitis, and many other conditions or maladies. The only negative to this protocol is the need for a technician to do the injection.

VIRILITY — Ozone Therapy is effective for both genders. Men seem to suffer more than women from this condition. Results vary based on age and severity, but most ED will go away after six or seven direct injections of 50 cc's or more. It takes twenty or more sessions (10 minutes) on the Breathing Apparatus to achieve the same result. However, once virility is reestablished, a daily session with the Breathing Apparatus will keep the male libido healthy. (A note of precaution — ED is usually a sign of a more serious condition which is usually circulation and heart related. Sometimes a mild stroke could have caused the ED. Get a check-up!)

Ladies who are postmenopausal have discovered the reverse aging properties of vaginals in regard to their sex drive, and that the use of ozonated oils augments the vaginals and direct injections. Applied topically to the penis or vagina, the ozonated oil will, in time, reduce the blockages and stimulate the libido (this takes months, folks). Using the oils in conjunction with Direct Injection, Vaginal Insufflation, or Breathing Apparatus, seems to be most effective. Several of my clients take ozonated honey in addition to using the breathing apparatus. They report excellent results. My personal experience with the breathing apparatus augmented with ozonated honey has been very positive.

VICE CONTROL — The Breathing Apparatus has been used by several clients to eliminate their nicotine addiction. It has worked seventy percent of the time. Willpower, stress, and the discipline to use the Breathing Apparatus seem to be the variables. I only have one client who is using the Breathing Apparatus to eliminate his dependency on alcohol. Vamos a ver, I hope we see some success with this application. Perhaps if we have some successes with these forms of vice control, we can then try others; specifically, drug addiction.

WEIGHT CONTROL — Listen to your common sense. Ozone therapy is not a magic bullet that will convert pies, cakes, donuts, potato chips and junk food into an athletic build or a bikini figure. Ozone therapy does increase one's energy level. If you use this energy for exercise and if metabolism is in sync with a healthy body and, if a diet is structured properly, then weight loss will occur. (Note all the *ifs.*)

CAUTION!
- •If you drink alcohol, you undo the positive effects of ozone therapy.
- •If you exercise directly after ozone therapy, you are mitigating the effects of your protocol by burning the added oxygen in your blood for muscle use rather than healing.
- •If you smoke after ozone therapy you will diminish the effect of your protocol.
- •Soda pop, greasy foods, junk foods? Do I really need to say anything?

CHAPTER 4a

HOW IT ALL WORKS

Nicola Tesla invented the ozone generator around 1900. He replicated nature by running oxygenated air through a glass tube and shocking the 02 (oxygen) molecules with high voltage. The 02 molecules split into two separate 01 molecules and shortly after leaving the chamber the 01 molecules reassembled in clusters of three, creating the element 03 — OZONE. This gas is unstable and wants to return to its 02 form -- back to OXYGEN.

Most modern ozone generators work on the same basic principle that Tesla created. They achieve 03 no matter what is used as a tube conductor — stainless steel, glass, ceramic, or crystal. The size of the tube and flow rate (length & circumference) normally determines the amount of 03 one receives. Other determiners are the oxygen source: pure oxygen or ambient air. The power supply is structured around transformers and electronics that produce around 3500 volts. Ozone is measured in grams per hour or portions thereof. Most generators (I've purchased a dozen.) have a rheostat to regulate the ozone output. I don't know why. No one, I repeat, NO ONE (not the manufacturers or so-called Experts) has ever explained why one would want less ozone than the machine can produce. I've taken all these generators apart and inspected and tested them. The dial is nothing more than a dimmer switch which reduces the electrical current to the transformer, thereby reducing the amount of 03 and allowing intermittent 02 to inhabit the output tube. Again — WHY? Varying the voltage is dangerous!

My inventions take a different approach. Most of the protocols that provide rapid cures for cancer, heart disease, strokes, and multiple sclerosis require direct injections to begin the cures, using vaginals and Breathing Apparatus to augment and prevent any healing erosion. In order to obtain a smooth injection, one has to have more than 03 with intermittent 02 molecules entering the bloodstream. (besides, that hurts like a dirty bugger) All the protocols require more than just 03. There are two - and only two - ozone generators on the market today that generate 06, 09, and sometimes 012. The

Brockman machine from Nogales and mine, the Old Tree. Brockman's two stage uses ultrasound to make the 03 molecules bond, creating 06 and 09. My machine uses a quartz modulator and a voltage variance to accomplish the

same 06, 09 and sometimes 012.

Which is the better machine?

I used the Brockman for years. I loved it until it became almost unavailable and expensive. (Three-year waiting list and a $5,000 price with a fifty percent deposit at the time of order.) That's what prompted me to delve into the industry and come up with a viable alternative. I believe, and so do others, that I've created an ozone generator that is perhaps a little better than the Brockman. Factor in the breathing apparatus I invented and there is none other close to being the same quality. Hands down, my system is far superior. Plus, my systems are available to ship

within thirty days and are priced at slightly under $4000. That price includes the Breathing Apparatus. (You can't buy the units separately unless you have one of my Old Tree model 06 generators.)

Let's discuss the basic science behind the breathing apparatus. The normal person, and the majority of doctors and some scientists, refer to the "smell of ozone". The climate change experts talk about the layers of ozone in the atmosphere. On local television stations they refer to the air pollution and talk about the ozone pollution level.

That's all talk - highly uneducated blather. OZONE HAS NO SMELL, TASTE or COLOR! As I mentioned above, Peter Brockman pointed this out to me years ago during a phone conversation, and I have proven it with my Breathing Apparatus!

When lightning strikes, you have been told you are smelling ozone. NOPE! That's nitric acid (HNO_3) you are smelling. When lightning (high voltage) splits the molecules of 02 into 01's, they regroup as 03 which is ozone. When ozone is mixed with the ambient air, it forms a variety of elements. Hydrogen, oxygen, nitrogen, carbon dioxide plus all the pollutants that are in the air, create a variety of elements and nitric acid is the most noxious. If you take pure 03 made from an ozone generator using medical grade oxygen, the substance you smell coming out of the tube is nitric acid. This acid will burn a neoprene glove and literally dissolve it if the ozone is strong like 06 or 09. HNO_3 is the element of nitric acid. I've devised a way to take away some of the H and some of the N and pass it through a device that uses no electricity. I use a variety of precious metals and my secret method to activate (excite)the molecules that neutralize some of the nitrogen and the hydrogen. The result is 06 or 09 in a form you can breathe. The toxic nitric acid had been eliminated. The

breathing apparatus is a major breakthrough in Ozone Therapy.

Chapter 5a

Protocols — Ozone Generator plus the Breathing apparatus.

- Straight mask breathing:
(On average, it has been estimated by users that one minute of deep breathing is comparable to one cc of direct injection.)
- Ear insufflation:
Never put the tube directly into the ear. No longer than five minutes per ear. The eardrum is a very sensitive membrane that can be damaged if you place nitric acid on it for any length of time. I'm working a device that may minimize this problem.
- Vaginal insufflation:
Fifteen minutes of vaginal insufflation is equal to approximately 45-50 CCs of direct injection.
- Sitz bath with warm water:
Remember, if you use a plastic tub, it may delaminate. Try to find an old galvanized wash tub — or something ceramic, like a bathtub.
- Rectal insufflation:
Not my favorite protocol; however, one should cleanse thoroughly with multiple enemas before doing the ozone.
- Water purification:
Thirty seconds for one liter if you use a stone. Perhaps a little longer if the water is questionable. Remember, the solids won't go away (mud). Use a filter before ozonating if possible.
- Ozonating oils for topical applications:
Palm oil and coconut oil are my preference for topical applications. For ingestion, it is the same, plus ozonated honey and cane syrup. Five minutes for every four ounces is sufficient for all medicated oils. Palm and coconut will harden if refrigerated. The effective life is ten days to three weeks, depending upon refrigeration or room temperature (refrigerated lasts longer).
Honey has to be heated to increase the viscosity before ozonating. Don't use a stone unless you like cleaning up a mess.
- Concentrated eye wash (water) for cataract treatment: Use water at room temperature — a small amount in a glass container. Ozonate for 5 minutes. The ozonation will heat the water to near body temperature. Use an eyewash cup or a shot glass to cleanse the open eye. Four to five minutes for each eye. Do the protocol immediately — twice a day if possible.
- Concentrated water or oil for gum disease:

Dental applications for gum disease should be injections directly in the tissue. It is painful. Have your dentist deaden the tissue before injections. Use ozonated coconut oil as a toothpaste and gum wash in between dental appointments.

- Ozonating water for vegetable and meat preparation: One or two minutes per liter will make your water almost medical grade. Wash the vegetables thoroughly and then place them in a bowl of ozonated water and refrigerate. Not only have you removed the pesticides, your veggies and fruits will stay fresh for many more days.

  Meats chicken,fish: wash in ozonated water, pat dry with paper towels and then refrigerate or freeze. Fruits should be washed and then dried if left at room temperature. Removing the pesticides from all food products will lengthen their shelf life and minimize your intake of toxins. Remember to always use stainless steel or glass.

  NO ALUMINUM OR PLASTIC!

Chapter 6a

Virility:

First, I need to describe my daily routine. I live alone. I eat healthy and use my ozone breathing apparatus every morning when the sun comes up and again in the afternoon. Not long — just ten minutes each session.

This breathing apparatus is my invention. It neutralizes the nitric acid and permits me to breathe straight ozone into my system. I have not had a direct injection of ozone since December 4, 2015, and only the use of my breathing apparatus.

I'm 74 and have a strong libido.

Seven years ago, I experienced a life changing health issue; a major HEART ATTACK!! Prognosis: The cardiologist recommended a triple bypass within a week or I was certain to die. I knew he was correct about dying if I let that clown cut into me and then use Panama's hospital system. NO THANKS! I went home and called Doctor Carl. He explained how to proceed.

So, I opted not to have a triple bypass and used ozone therapy to cure the heart condition. Within two months of having this life-threatening occurrence, my libido improved drastically. I could relate details, but it will sound like an old man bragging. Ozone Therapy with my protocols, works. I have testimonials from many men who have experienced this turn-around.

The point I'm trying to make is very simple. A man's virility is important on several levels including physical gradations and mental health. The older one gets; the more important libido is to the male psyche. Overall health begins to deteriorate when a man experiences ED, which is usually a sign that something else is wrong with his health. The psychological impact is heavy. When ED strikes, many men begin to give up, drink heavily, and compound the condition. The flip side is the search for the magic elixir such as the ground rhino horn, the puffer fish poison gland, the voodoo spell. These attitudes usually result in some form of chemical inducement — legal and/or illegal. One doesn't need to be an expert to know these substances are not curing but are ultimately harming an existing condition.

Let me explain how ozone therapy cures ED. Male erections are created by blood flow. If your circulation system is clogged or restricted, blood will not flow to that region and you remain flaccid. Ozone therapy — specifically the direct injection protocol- begins cleaning veins, arteries, and capillaries so that you not only are you regaining your libido, you are age reversing your overall health. As the circulatory system begins to flow freely, blood pressure goes down, veins and arteries begin to soften and become malleable again — in effect your libido becomes young again. Once a man can obtain an erection by experiencing female stimulus, he no longer needs the direct injection if the breathing apparatus is available. My ozone system, common sense and a good diet is sufficient to maintain that youthful libido.

Chapter 7a

Summary and recommendations

Often, I receive criticism for not engaging with the medical profession with my inventions, knowledge, and experience. Perhaps I deserve some of the negatives because of my anti-medical attitude.

I'm not against doctors or hospitals. I'm against the ignorance, attitude, and conceit they have propagated toward alternative medicine. Unfortunately, one cannot go anywhere within the medical community and discuss a system that sells for less than five thousand dollars and can provide medical miracles and anti-aging for an entire family or neighborhood. The idea is preposterous to their way of thinking — plus if it is acknowledged then the medical community will suffer tremendous financial setbacks, especially the pharmaceutical companies.

My attitude regarding conventional mainline medicine is this: I'll let you set my broken leg, dig out the bullet from a gunshot wound, remove my appendix if necessary, and even let you diagnose a life-threatening malady. I'll listen to your recommendations but color me skeptical when you tell me you can cure my major malady — like my heart attack or a stroke or cancer. I'll let you run your tests, examine my bodily fluids, but YOU AIN'T GONNA CUT ON ME until I look at every alternative, including voodoo!

****

Recommended equipment and supplies for a home or family Ozone System.

- Old Tree Model 06 Ozone Generator which includes a 03 Breathing Apparatus. (tubing and fitting are included in the package — as well as a couple of stones for ozonating water and oils)
- A medical oxygen tank and regulator, <u>OR</u> an oxygen concentrator that uses molecular sieve technology. Or both. A small medical oxygen tank for injections, and the oxygen concentrator for all other protocols.
- A 50 ml (cc) glass syringe
- A tourniquet of some kind.
- A box of neoprene gloves (for testing ozone strength)
- #23 butterfly needles
- Cotton balls and alcohol
- A large package of individually wrapped drinking straws. These sanitary and disposable straws are used for vaginals and ozonating oils and honey.
- Oxygen masks for breathing apparatus

For further information, questions, or discussion contact me directly.
Robert Hatting -- <u>bobhatting@gmail.com</u>